STARBRIGHT

MEDITATIONS FOR CHILDREN

STARBRIGHT

MEDITATIONS FOR CHILDREN

Maureen Garth

HarperSanFrancisco

A Division of HarperCollinsPublishers

FIRST U.S. EDITION

Library of Congress Cataloging-in-Publication Data

Garth, Maureen.
    Starbright: meditations for children/Maureen Garth.—1st U.S. ed.
        p.   cm.
    Summary: Describes the methods and positive effects of meditation
and presents a collection of brief meditations.
    ISBN 0-06-250398-7 (alk. paper)
    1. Meditations—Juvenile literature.   2. Meditation—Juvenile literature.
[1. Meditations. 2. Meditation.] I. Title.
BL624.2.G37 1991
158'.12'083—dc20   90–56458
                                          CIP
                                          AC

    93   94   95   96   97   CWI   10 9 8 7 6 5 4

This edition is printed on acid-free paper that meets the American National Standards Institute Z39.48 Standard.

Contents

Introduction

Why I Started Meditations
with my Daughter

I began doing meditations with my daughter, Eleanor, when she was around three years of age, just simple ones that enabled her to have a peaceful night. She had always slept well, although there were a couple of occasions when she almost certainly had nightmares. She became distressed, and this may have prompted the idea of meditation. I enjoy meditating and felt that by using this means of expression, I could create a tranquil night transition from activity into peace for Eleanor.

I started with very simple ideas, like giving her an imaginary companion so that she would feel protected and never alone. I told

Eleanor that from the time we are born we each have a protector who watches over us and who loves us. I gave this guardian angel really large golden wings to wrap around Eleanor so that she would always feel secure.

At such an early age children need the reassurance of always being cared for, as the night and the dark can be very scary. Later I added to the guardian a garden that gave Eleanor somewhere to go in her dreams, a place that was peaceful and where she felt secure.

When Eleanor was four, I gave her a star to focus on. Often I would make it a pink star (her favorite color); sometimes it would be any other color that took my fancy. At other times I would give the star speckles or perhaps stripes. I did whatever I thought would appeal to the imagination of a child.

To enable her to relax, I filled the star with white light, which I brought down through the top of her head, into her arms, hands, and fingers, down the trunk, and into the legs, feet, and toes. Children find this an easy exercise in visualization, as stars are important to them. If you look at children's drawings, stars and suns appear with regularity. Not so the moon, a fact that is interesting, because they speak about it and point it out as though it were the most fascinating thing they had ever seen. Yet the moon rarely appears in their drawings, whereas six-pointed stars and huge glowing suns often do.

I started to embellish Eleanor's time in the garden by giving her a tree house, taking her behind waterfalls, going to her own pool where the animals drank, and so on. I let my imagination run free and I found that I too was thoroughly enjoying the meditations. I loved it when I made her small and gave her fairy wings or did other things that I felt would be special for her imagination.

Eleanor is now eight and her star is very important to her. She is most unhappy if I say I am too tired or busy (which does not happen often), but she can do a meditation for herself. She does not need me to do it for her, but she loves the comfort and the closeness of my being there and doing it with her. In fact, she now tells me a story before I do her meditation, and her storytelling is delightful.

Sharing with Friends

I often have children over to stay, which means that they share in Eleanor's star—only of course, it becomes their own special star. Why wouldn't they have something special to them and only to them? Their imaginations roam as they have different-colored stars, multicolored stars, or perhaps just one beautiful silver star that sparkles and shimmers with glorious light.

I have found that this star has become very important to many of Eleanor's friends. It delights them when I tuck them in at night with a loving kiss and hug and then, while their eyes are tightly shut, speak quietly to them of the wonders the star brings. Then I take them on a journey through fantasy-land. I have had children ask, even if they haven't stayed with us for a year or so, "Will you do that special thing you did the last time?" They remember it because their experience was beautiful and their imagination was stirred.

Some of the children have told me they have seen "space," and they describe it well; some have seen "other worlds," some castles or gold at the end of the rainbow, and so on. It is interesting to listen to them and to see the enjoyment they have gained from being quiet even for such a short period of time. When the meditations are done at nighttime you let them drift into sleep. Come morning, they love to relate what they saw and did. They do not always remember, but they do have a good peaceful sleep.

How Meditation Helps Children

Unfortunately, a lot of children have trouble learning these techniques by the time they are seven or eight. Relaxation and visualization, if taught at an earlier age, could enhance not only children's school work but other areas of their lives. Their concentration would improve; their artistic abilities would develop; they would feel more centered; their daydreaming could not only bring joy, but be constructive.

I have become aware of the quality of my daughter's written stories, the way she uses her imagination and the creativity of her text. Her choice of words is unusual and effective: "_they were swifting by so firm and nice", "_she said in a sorrowful sulk", "_they said in silent voices."

Her stories include not only fairies and "little" people but also real people, travel in shells, rainbows, and so on. Perhaps she would have had this unusual quality of expression regardless of the star, but maybe her star helped to release her imagination.

Although I am giving what I hope is a good selection of meditations in this book, they are only examples. It is more important for you to let *your* imagination roam where it will, and come up with thoughts and scenes particularly special to you and yours. Do not restrict yourself: let it all flow and you will be amazed, not only at how easy it is, but at how much pleasure you gain from the scenes that you are creating.

In this way you are forming a bond with your children that can be passed along to their children, and so on. You may thus help future generations to be more aware and more centered than we were.

Another thing I do is to fill children's hearts with love. Sometimes I "make" their hearts large and pulsating so that they can feel the extent of the love they are putting out to other children or to adults or to the animals. Some children see a door going into their hearts that they unlock and then go inside. It is wonderful to open the way, for some children at least, to be able to express the love they feel when they unlock that door.

How to Begin

Each meditation starts with the star, the focal point for setting up the conditions for the meditation. Indeed, it is an integral part, as this is where the relaxation and visualization starts. The star is followed by the angel, which in turn can be followed by the Worry Tree (if you feel it is necessary), and then you do the meditation you have selected, that is, the Grandfather Tree, the fairies, or any of the other meditations. Do whatever you feel is appropriate to the mood of the child or children, or even yourself.

Although I used a star as the focal point, you might prefer to use the moon or the sun. It does not matter which; the important thing is to give your child something to focus on. For relaxation and visualization, it is as easy to bring the light down from the sun or moon as a star.

If you use the moon, for instance, you could say that the moon's fingers are spreading out over the world so that everyone can see in the night, but there is one special moonbeam that is coming down just for your child. That moonbeam is filled with glitter, little sprinkles of which are touching all parts of the body, making it glow.

If it is the sun you have selected, you could speak about how the sun is a golden ball in the sky, filled with warmth and light. A large shaft of sunshine is dancing down to the child's bed, where it is caressing and embracing her or him, filling every part of the body. *You* must choose the vehicle with which you feel the most at ease, be it the sun, moon, or the star.

Again the same applies to the guardian angel theme. You must feel comfortable with what you are saying. You might prefer to use another descriptive mode: a protective guardian who could appear as a very wise older person who throws a gold cloak around the child to provide security.

For the Parents

If you do not feel at home with what you are doing, you may have difficulty imparting the feeling that goes with the meditations. What I have written need not be taken literally. If you were to select the Grandfather Tree and put it into your own words, that would be fine. The meditations included here are simply examples of what could be said. You could make up your own by speaking of your child's favorite things or activities. If your child is very interested in trains, for instance, you could either put him or her into a train that is winding its way through the countryside, or you could indeed make the child the eyes and ears of the train to experience the feelings of the train moving along. Or you could place your child on a magic carpet that flies over the cities and the mountains, giving a fantastic vantage point. *What* is said depends very much upon you, the parent, and the individual child. The most important thing is the warmth and intimacy engendered by your spending this quiet time with your child, a time that is different from that spent in reading.

For Teachers

At my daughter's school I have done meditations for the eight-year-old children. It was quite noticeable that the children who learned more easily were able to concentrate and to visualize what I was saying, while the ones who had learning problems fidgeted and could not settle. Meditation or visualization could be very constructive in harnessing the thoughts of children who tend to scatter their energies in directions that are not productive.

As well as doing the meditations at Riley Street Infants School, Sydney, I also helped with the children's "publishing," which proved to be a lot of fun. The difference in what they wrote from the time the meditations were started was noticeable. Most children used to write fairly short stories. The content was generally about their families or something happening around them. Later their stories became longer and the content more detailed, and they were based less in the here and now and more in the world of fantasy. The expression also greatly improved.

The meditations in this book can be used in the daytime, though they have been written more in a nighttime mode. You will find that I always leave the children in the garden, or on a cloud, or wherever, as I want them to drift into sleep happily. Obviously you cannot do this in a classroom or if you are teaching a group of children during the day.

In the daytime you would take them to the spot in the meditation where you felt they would settle and say: "I am going to be very quiet now and leave you for a while. Go where you will, because you are very safe and I will bring you back shortly." Leave them in their meditation for five or ten minutes, according to their attention span, then bring them back out of the garden, gently closing the gate behind them. Take them past the Worry Tree, where they have left all their problems, and tell them to open their eyes when they are ready.

After doing your meditation, you will find it interesting to ask each child what he or she saw. The ones whose concentration is good settle into a calm and tranquil state that is beautiful to behold. They like to share their experiences, while the ones who have difficulty will have little or nothing to relate. But if you persevere for a time, you will find that the restless ones will start to settle, to see things, and to fidget less. Remarkably, their school work will improve, because they are learning the art of concentration.

Boys and Girls

Because many boys have been raised to believe that "only girls do things like that," they thought that meditation was silly. It is unfortunate that their more empathetic qualities are not brought out; rather they are taught that their "feminine" qualities are to be overcome in order to preserve their masculinity. Little has been done to encourage them to reach their full potential by having honest feelings. They would be much happier if they could express their emotions freely and without fear of ridicule. The meditations in this book could help to release some of the limitations that society has imposed on boys at such an early age, and therefore enable them to lead happier and more productive lives.

In the last meditation of the school year I really wanted to introduce fairies, elves, and dancing, but I was unsure how eight-year-old boys would react. However, I felt a strong urge to do it, and with great trepidation, off I went. I was agreeably surprised to find how much the boys enjoyed the meditation and amazed when the greatest skeptic of all said: "That's the best one yet."

Eleanor's class was a mixed one, and I found that both the boys and girls enjoyed whatever meditation or story I made up. In every class there are always a few timid children, and, although I would suggest that you emphasize the fact that nothing in the garden is harmful and that even the largest animal is tame, you could always do a story where the child is brave and strong, setting off alone in the garden not knowing what might be encountered. However, I would still stress the fact that they are protected and that no harm can befall them.

Problem Children

Those children who had difficulty with the concept of meditation, not having been exposed to it, also had poor concentration and found it difficult to sit for any length of time. Children love stories, and the practice of reading regularly to them each night is an aid to their concentration. This requires effort and perserverance, especially for working parents who have little time or perhaps in a family that is too large for much individual attention.

With the "problem" children I would spend time talking, individually, in order to explain what meditation is and how we would go about it. I was concerned at first that singling them out might make them feel insecure, but rather it gave a lift to their fragile egos

and made them feel important. During the next meditation, I would place these children close to me, because I found that my nearness seemed to help them to drift off peacefully.

I did not draw attention to the fact they did not settle easily or that they did not see anything. I would ask them why they seemed to find it difficult. Inevitably it would be that they did not understand what they were supposed to do nor how they were meant to "see" and needed more guidance. I would explain that as I spoke I wanted them to "see" my words form pictures in their minds and that if they did not see the pictures I was describing, they might see something that I could not and they might care to tell me about it afterward.

I have found the Worry Tree (see page 20) essential when doing meditations at the school. Often the children who cannot settle have problems at home, perhaps with parents, perhaps with siblings. Because the problems could be related to school, or to their friends, it is good to set up a Worry Tree where they can pin their worries before entering the peace of their garden. When they return from their garden, they certainly will not want to pick up their worries and bring them back into their everyday life.

The Tone of Voice

You might think, when you read the meditations, that they are not very long. Please remember that when you are speaking, you will do so in a very slow, relaxed voice, pausing to let the scene sink in, so that the child, whose eyes are closed and who is focusing inward, can easily visualize and feel the scene. The way you use your voice is very important. You will find it best to drop your voice by a few tones, speaking more and more slowly, with a soothing quality. There is something hypnotic about a voice that is low and relaxed.

Some of the meditations are longer than others. If you are tired, then select a short one. I have found that the children are not concerned with the length, only with the fact that *you* are doing it for *them*.

Although I call them meditations, you might prefer to call them stories. This really is not important; it is only a name. The main thing is that you will be sharing a unique experience with your very special child.

What is Meditation?

Meditation is a time for reflection and contemplation—a time to go within. It is not beyond the reach of anyone, provided they take the time and create the opportunity for it. Meditation is very simple; it means sitting quietly either on your own or with a group of people (it is best to sit in an upright chair—if you make the chair too comfortable, you may fall asleep). It is preferable to wear loose clothing for comfort, but if that is not possible, loosen anything that is tight around the waist or neck so that you do not feel these restrictions. It is wise not to cross your arms or legs, as this can lead to discomfort.

You might like to have soothing music in the background or you might prefer silence. Sometimes I like to fix a scene in my head, such as the garden in which I place the children. Other times my mind is like a blank screen ready to receive whatever images happen to cross it. It is up to the individual to decide how long to spend in meditation. If you can spare only five or ten minutes that can be ample. However, to feel the full benefit, twenty minutes is better, because meditation can promote calmness, relax tension, and give relief from anxiety as you become detached from your problems. Your problems will not necessarily go away, but meditation can be beneficial to the way you handle those problems. Sometimes the solution comes when we take the time to sit quietly. Meditation is a very soothing, relaxing way of coping with the stress and anxiety of daily life. Many doctors recommend meditation for their patients as a wise and good practice. It is a very relaxing and pleasant way to spend such a short period of time, and one that has many benefits.

This book is being written for several reasons, the main one being to give pleasure to children. Meditation has been so much a part of our own lives that it gives me great joy to share it with others. I also believe in the need for society to look at different ways of bonding, and I am hopeful that this book will fill that need.

I hope you enjoy the meditations as much as the children do, and I trust that the peace and harmony they produce will flow around you and yours.

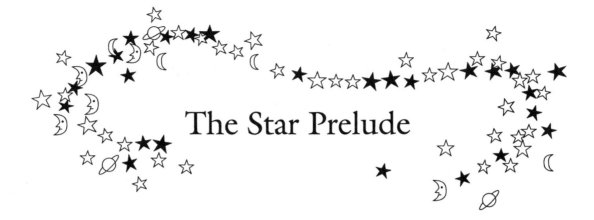

The Star Prelude

I WANT you to see above your head a beautiful, beautiful star. This star is very special to you, as it is your very own star. It can be any color you like—you might see it as being a purple star, or perhaps a pink one—or blue—or yellow—or is it a speckled star? Or a silver one? Because it is your very own star, it can be any color or colors you choose.

This special star is filled with white light, lovely

white light that shimmers and glows. I want you to see this light streaming down toward you until it reaches the very top of your head. And now I want you to bring this pure light down through your head and take it right down your body until your whole body is filled with this glorious white light.

I want you to feel the light going down your arms, right down, until you feel it reaching your hands and going into each and every finger.

Feel that light going down the trunk of your body, down until it reaches your legs, and when you feel it there, take it right down until it comes to your feet and then feel the light going through each toe.

I now want you to look into your heart and to

fill your heart with love for all the people and animals in the world. They are your friends, be they small or large. Can you see your heart getting bigger and bigger? It's expanding because you have so much love in your heart for all these people and the animals, and of course for yourself.

Now your guardian angel is waiting to wrap golden wings of protection around you before taking you into your garden. The angel's wings are very large and very soft, just like down. Everyone has their own guardian angel and that guardian angel takes care of you and protects you always, so you are never alone. It's important to remember this and to know that you have someone who looks after you with love and care.

Your guardian angel is now going to take you to a garden that is your own special place, but before you enter I want you to look at the large tree that is outside. This tree is called the Worry Tree. I want you to pin on this tree anything that might worry you—perhaps you have had some arguments at school or maybe you are having difficulty with your school work. This tree will take any worries at all, be it with your friends or your family. This tree accepts anything that you would care to pin there.

Your guardian angel is now opening the gate for you to enter, and as you go in you find the colors are like nothing you have seen before. The beauty of the flowers, the colors, the textures, and the perfume—breathe them in. The grass is a vivid green and the sky a beautiful blue with little white fluffy clouds. It is very peaceful in your garden; it is full of love and harmony.

> You may feel this prelude is very long, but it is wise to create with care, thought, and feeling the setting your child is entering. When your child is used to it, the prelude may become shorter, as it is not always necessary to describe the star and the angel in such full detail. Then it becomes something like the shorter version below.

I want you to see above your head a beautiful, beautiful star. This star is filled with lovely white light. I want you to bring the white light from that star right down through your body until you can feel it in every part of your body, and your heart is filled with love for all humanity and for all creatures great and small.

Your guardian angel is waiting for you to wrap a golden cloak of protection around you and take you to the Worry Tree. Put anything that worries you on the tree, and then your guardian will open the gate and take you inside your garden.

Your garden is filled with glorious flowers; the grass and the trees are an emerald green, and the sky a deep blue with little white clouds.

After you have set the scene, as it were, you can do anything with the children that you think they would enjoy. Become a child again yourself—I think you will be surprised at the pleasure these flights of fantasy will give you.

Some of the meditations I have done follow.

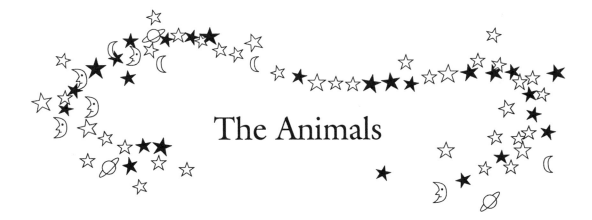

The Animals

As YOU walk down the path in your special garden, you feel the warmth of the sun caressing you. There is a very gentle breeze blowing, and you can hear the birds calling to each other. There is nothing in your garden that can harm you; each and every creature lives in harmony with the others.

I want you to feel the peace that is flowing in your garden and the gentleness of all who live there.

Your path is winding through the trees, and it will take you to a water hole where all the animals come to drink. When you go down to the water's edge you will find the animals coming over to say "hello" to you.

There are tortoises who are very slow and ponderous and love the feel of the sun on their shells. The proud white swans go by gracefully, while the ducks make lots of noise. Now you can see some deer coming down to drink, and walking with them are lions and tigers. You can pat them when they reach you and give them a big cuddle, as all these creatures love being cuddled. In your garden there are no fierce animals because they have no reason to be afraid, and neither have you.

The hippopotamuses are having a lovely time washing themselves and each other with the water, and now the elephants are joining in. I think you should step into the water and swim with them. If you feel a little tired, you can climb on the back of the elephant and let it hose you down.

I can see the giraffes coming to drink. If you get out of the water now, I am sure you can have a ride on the back of one of them. Yes, you are getting onto the giraffe's back now and off you go. Because you are sitting up so high, you can see into the trees, and it is wonderful to be able to do this. You can stroke the kangaroos and look into their pouches, very gently of course, and there's a squirrel—isn't it a busy little creature.

I am going to leave you now to explore your garden with your newfound friends. If you want to get off the giraffe's back and go by foot, that's all right. Perhaps you might decide to ride on a tiger for a change.

There is so much to see and do, and I know you will have a lovely, lovely time . . .

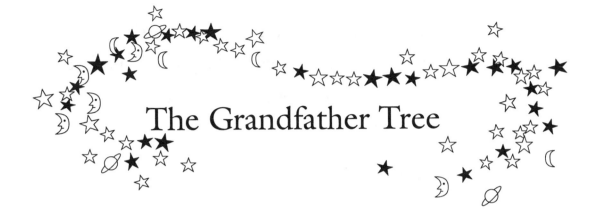

The Grandfather Tree

THE AIR is so fresh and clean, the perfume of the flowers is rich, and the sun a huge golden ball, sending down a very gentle heat. The trees are waving their arms in welcome—they have been waiting for you to come into your special garden, and the trees want to talk to you. If you listen you can hear them saying: "Come to me, come to me."

There is one tree that stands out from the

others. He is very, very old. He is the grandfather of all the trees, and he is full of knowledge and wisdom. There is nothing this tree doesn't know. He has been watching what happens around him ever since he was a young sapling.

He has a very thick trunk and big, big roots going out through the earth. As they go down into the depths of the earth, these roots push the earth up, making mounds big enough to sit on. This Grandfather Tree has plenty of branches with beautiful green leaves, so many leaves it's a wonder he can hold the branches as high in the air as he does.

The breeze is rustling the grass and the leaves on the trees are making sounds that are like the purest music one could imagine.

I want you to walk up to the Grandfather Tree. As you approach the trunk of this tree, you will see there is a door with a little handle. I want you to open this door and go inside. Close the door quietly behind you now, and you will find the inside of the tree is lit with a golden glow. In this glow, you can see passageways going through the branches. There is also another pathway going down the trunk into the roots.

Why don't you go and investigate? You have plenty of time to choose which way to go. I wonder what you will find? I think there are rooms off these passageways that hold all sorts of knowledge. Some have lots of toys. There are always people around to keep you company whom you can talk to. They will be able to answer your questions. If you want to remain on your own, you only have to say so and you can go into the room of your choice and do the things you most want to do.

I shall now leave you to explore your special tree . . .

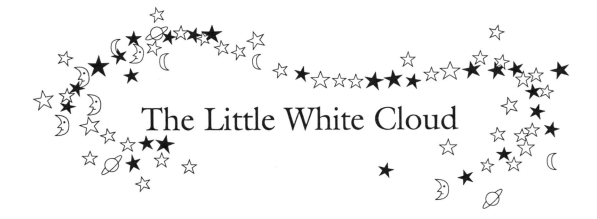

The Little White Cloud

YOUR guardian angel is closing the gate behind you, and your garden is beautiful. The colors are so rich and luxuriant, with that deep blue sky and the sun a radiant golden ball. And there are perky white clouds floating by.

As you go down your garden path, you will find that one of the white clouds has come down from the sky to take you for a ride. I want you to

climb on to this cloud. It is lovely and fluffy—
perhaps it's made of cotton wool? Or is it made out
of cotton candy? Look, there is a little seat with a set
of leather reins. You don't have to tell this cloud
where to go as it floats off into the wide blue sky.
Your cloud knows where it is going.

Now you are leaving the planet Earth behind.
I want you to look below. You will see Earth like a
gigantic ball with many different patterns. You can
see that these are the forests, the rivers, and the
mountains. The clusters of buildings are the cities,
and they are tightly packed in, but where the sheep,
horses, and cattle graze, there are only a few
buildings and barns. If you look VERY closely you can
see your home way, way below you.

And off you go, up and up, floating very peacefully on your soft downy cloud. The higher you go, the smaller Earth will appear to you, until it becomes just a speck in the distance. Have a good look around. You will see other small clouds that have children just like you who have been brought from their gardens to feel the freedom of floating in the heavens.

These little clouds are now stopping at a very large cloud. You can step off now and go for a walk on this big cloud. The other children are getting off too. You will find there are people there who like living in the clouds. They are called the Cloud People, and they wear flowing white robes with fluffy shoes and hats. The Cloud People love showing off their land of clouds to children—grown-ups are only sometimes invited, and then only if they have the right kind of imagination.

There is so much to do on this cloud. You certainly won't fall off, even if you hang over the side by the tips of your toes, because they have a different law of gravity in Cloudland. There are slippery dips and swings and roundabouts to ride. You can even go swimming in the cloud pool, which is all white and foamy.

What fun you can have here, so I think I will leave you now . . .

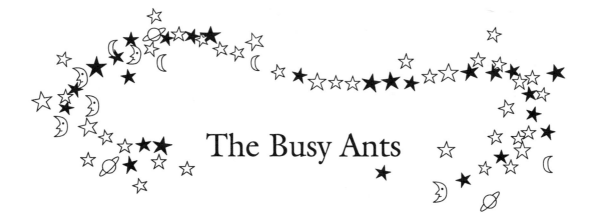

The Busy Ants

YOUR garden is so peaceful tonight. It is quiet, so quiet you can hear the ants moving around in the grass and on the trees. The air is crystal clear and fresh, and there is a very gentle breeze. I want you to feel that breeze caressing your cheeks and touching your hair.

Can you see the ants? They are always busy, working away so quietly. You could become the size of an ant if you wanted. I think that would be fun.

I want you now to become very, very small—see yourself shrinking in size until you are no bigger than an ant. The grass seems very tall now that you are small and each blade of grass is much higher than you are. There is dew on the blades and—plop! You have just had a bath.

The ants are so busy tonight, you could perhaps help them carry the food to their homes. They would appreciate your help, as there is so much for them to do. They carry their food in their mouths but they are giving you a basket, which makes it easier for you to carry things.

When they have finished their work, the ants are going to a party. You are invited to share in their fun and there will be lots of games. I know that you will like what they are going to eat. They have special fruit and berries that are laid out on green leaves, and a drink made of nectar that will slide down your throat.

Not many people are invited to their parties, but you are their friend and special. They are looking forward to you being with them. In fact, I think the party is really a special occasion because you are visiting them. They want you to meet as many of their families as you can.

I shall now leave you with the ants and their party . . .

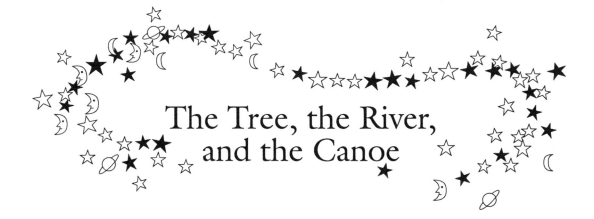

The Tree, the River,
and the Canoe

IN YOUR garden you will feel the warmth of the golden sun going through your body. There is a very gentle breeze, and the sky is a beautiful sapphire blue.

As you walk down your path you will come to a very old, gnarled tree. His branches are laden with leaves and they are moving gently in the light wind.

I want you to go to this tree and put your arms around the trunk so that you can feel in yourself the strength and life force of this tree. Feel the warmth of the earth coming up through your feet and meeting the life force of the tree. As you do this, you will feel a love for the earth and nature.

When you have finished hugging the tree, say "good-bye." Tell him that you will see him later on, but you want to go now to talk to the river. He is nodding his head in agreement and, if you look at his trunk, you will see a smile.

Off you go now, down to the river. The river is flowing very peacefully, and the water is so clear you can see right to the bottom. If you want, you can paddle your feet while you watch the golden fish swim by nibbling at their dinner.

I can see lots of canoes on the river. One is coming ashore for you—I can see you getting in. You don't have to paddle the canoe unless you want to, you can just lie back and relax as the waves gently rock the boat. Feel the warmth of the sun on your body.

As you drift down the stream, you notice little bridges crossing from one side to the other.

These bridges are arched over the water and they have red and yellow balloons floating from the center. A few of these balloons have fallen into the water. If you are quick, you could catch some before they drift away. There are people on these bridges and they are waving to you as you float past. Perhaps you may want to land your boat and explore. You could cross one of these bridges to see what's on the other side—or you may prefer to keep on drifting.

I shall leave you now in your canoe . . .

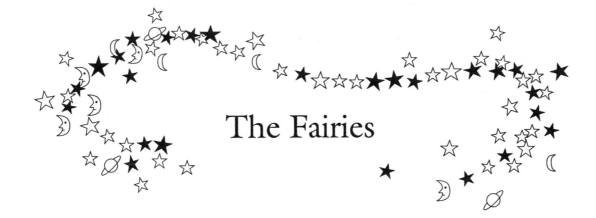

The Fairies

IN YOUR garden, the sky is a deep indigo blue with huge ballooning white clouds floating by and a yellow ball for the sun, it is so lovely and peaceful. You can see before you a pathway that is winding in and out of the trees. I want you to walk down that path until you come to a small clearing—if you look very, very carefully you can see the fairies. They have been waiting very patiently for you.

I want you to see yourself becoming smaller and smaller until you are just the same size as the fairies and the elves. They are very excited to have you visit them and they have made you a fantastic costume in your favorite color, and it glistens and glows in the sunlight. The fabric is so light it could float away if you didn't hold on to it.

To go with this magical outfit is a pair of wings that sparkle and shimmer in the sunlight. They are in a lighter shade than your costume. I want you now to dress up and put your wings on—and don't you look wonderful. The fairies are giving you a crown of flowers and herbs, and the perfume from these is rich and exciting.

The fairies want you to go flying with them,

and they will take you to examine the flowers that they look after. Each fairy has its own special flower and the perfume and clothes reflect its color and scent. When the fairies take off together, it's like looking at all the colors of the rainbow.

Two of the fairies, one on either side, will help you to fly, because this is the first time you have used your wings. It feels glorious to be free in the air. It's as though you were floating. They are taking you to their special flowers. You will land on the petals, which feel like velvet. If you lie down you will feel the softness of these petals and the sun warming the flowers.

When you have finished looking at the flowers, and you feel it's time to rest—after all, flying can be very tiring—I want you to come back to the clearing. The fairies and the elves are having a party for you. There will be fairy cookies, fairy bread, and gingerbread cakes. You will sit on a small toadstool with a bigger toadstool for a table, and you will drink from tiny pink shells.

There are many games to play, and I know you will enjoy playing with these little people . . .

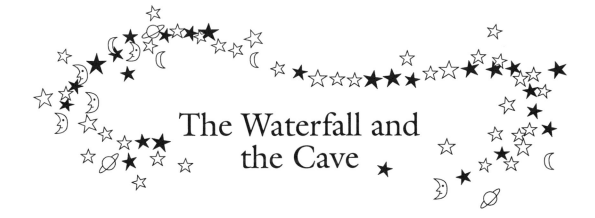

The Waterfall and the Cave

YOUR garden is full of interesting things tonight. I want you to take your skipping rope and to skip down the path on your way to the river. You can stop to speak to the deer and bunny rabbits, but don't stay too long. When you reach the river, you can watch the boats sailing by and people swimming as they enjoy themselves in the water.

They are having such a good time. I can hear their laughter. I can feel their happiness. Some of them are playing with a ball. I am sure if you wanted, you could join in too.

The river bank is a rich dark green. A line of weeping willow trees shades it with low slung branches trailing into the water. As you walk along the river's edge, you will come to a bend.

You cannot see around the bend yet, but as you walk on, you will see before you a high splashing waterfall. Drops of water are flying through the air and catching the sun's rays. They look like shining jewels in many colors and shapes. The falling water is creating a musical harmony that is rich and deep. From the bottom of the waterfall rises a cloud of misty spray.

If you climb to the side of the waterfall and look carefully, you will see there is an entrance to a passage behind the wall of water. You need sharp eyes to see the opening. Not many people would be aware it was there. I think you should find out what secrets it holds.

As you go behind the spray and into the entrance, you find that you are now in a large light cave. The water is falling down in front of you in a great thundering stream that seems to increase the silence in the cave. You can see through the water to watch what's happening on the other side, though no one there can see you.

As you look around, you will notice there are drawings on the walls. These have been here for many, many years. They must have been drawn by the Waterfall People who lived here such a long time ago.

As you look, you see passageways going off in different directions from the sides and the back of your cave. Why don't you walk down one of these passages to see what you can find? It's like going on a treasure hunt. I feel sure you will bring back many wonderful things . . .

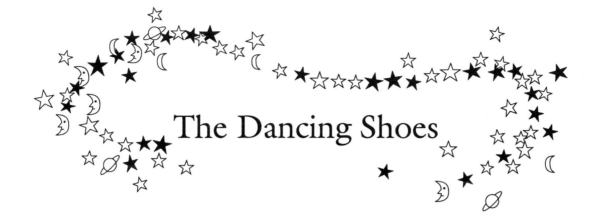

The Dancing Shoes

THE SKY is so clear, there isn't a cloud. The warmth of the sun radiates toward the earth and to where you are in your garden.

There is an air of excitement, as the "little" people have been waiting for you to come. They have been so very patient and they have kept themselves busy getting everything ready for you—

can you hear the music? There are stringed instruments playing and I can hear a harp.

Together they make music that is heavenly, music such as you have never heard before, the sort of music that makes you want to dance and dance.

Of course the "little" people already know this, and they have made you a special pair of dancing shoes. These dancing shoes are little red ones with sparkles on them. They have a bow across the top, and the heel is just the right size. These shoes are magic dancing shoes. Whoever wears them can dance and dance, never wanting to stop while the music plays.

I want you now to dance for all the people. While you twist and twirl, listen to the music and feel it deep inside yourself. You are having such a good time that you feel you might never stop dancing. Your energy is high and you like having an audience.

When you decide you have had enough, you can rest underneath a huge mushroom and watch the festivities from there. The mushroom is like a giant umbrella shading you from the sun. The grass underneath feels like a soft green cushion that you can sink into. Perhaps you want to take your shoes off for a while, although they look so pretty on your feet you may want to keep them on.

You might want to do some more dancing, or maybe it's time to see what's happening under the other mushrooms. Why don't you take a walk and see what's going on . . .

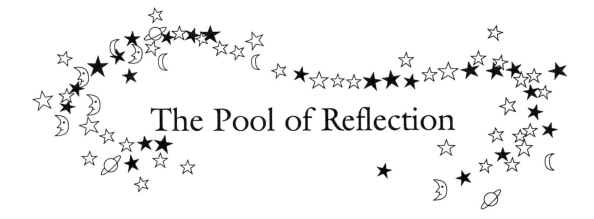

The Pool of Reflection

I CAN hear the birds twittering tonight. They are very busy as they get ready for bed. The nightingale is singing his own special song for you. You know, the nightingales sing the most beautiful melodies. The squirrels have finished gathering their nuts, the ants have taken their food home, and the bees have taken the pollen to their queen. The wise owls sit on the branches with their eyes wide open, the frogs are croaking in the nearby creek, and, there, I see a ginger kitten with her mother being taught how to look after herself. There are lots of animals in your garden tonight, and they like to play together.

As you walk through your garden, listening to all this activity, you will come to a very large pool. I want you to go to this pool and look very deeply into it. First you will see your own reflection. Then the ripples will take it away and the water will be smooth like glass.

This is the Pool of Reflection. I want you to go down into these special waters—you don't need goggles or a mask as you would in ordinary water. In the Pool of Reflection you can breathe as easily as if you were on land. When you feel the waters closing above your head, open your eyes. Down in the pool, it is bright and the moon shines into the cool green water. You will see fish of every imaginable color swimming every which way. There are rainbow fish in abundance.

There are trout, dogfish, and even catfish, but it is the rainbow fish that really catch your eye. Their colors glisten and gleam in the clean waters of your special pool.

When you look around you will notice colored coral everywhere. It glows pink in the moonlight that filters down through the waters, throwing up the different shades and highlighting the brilliant hues and strange shapes of the coral.

As you go further down, you will meet the large fish of the sea—the whales, the dolphins, and the sharks. They are all playing happily together. There is nothing to fear in this beautiful pool, and they are all friends.

When you reach the bottom of this pool, you will find houses made of sand. They have no doors, nor indeed is there glass in the windows. Their garden is made out of seaweed that moves with the current of the water. There are many shells in the garden, and some tiny sea creatures live in these shells.

The Water People live here and they can float in and out of their homes as they want. They love the peace and quiet at the bottom of this pool, and they would love to have you stay with them for a while. They can show you a different life from what you already know, so why don't you drift off with them . . .

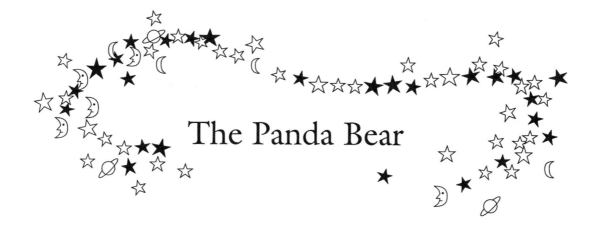

The Panda Bear

THE AIR is fresh and clean in your garden; the sun is sending out gentle rays that touch your body and make you feel good. The sky has lots of small clouds, and the birds are calling to each other.

The green of the trees and the grass is very lush, and there are bluebells and roses in all the rosy colors. Scattered between these flowers are brilliant yellow daisies nodding their heads in the gentle breeze.

There is someone waiting for you in your garden, someone who is very patient. I wonder if you know who it is? Why don't you go down your favorite path, then go behind the wise old tree and have a look. Perhaps someone is playing hide-and-seek—why don't you look quickly around the other side of the tree.

And there he is! A BIG black and white panda is waiting to give you a BIG cuddle. Why don't you climb onto his lap and put your arms around him, and then you will feel the warmth of his fur on your skin. This panda loves being cuddled and holding children close—he is holding out some bamboo for you to eat, so why don't you try some?

Panda Bear has lots of things to tell you that are secrets. He might tell you where he has left Mrs. Panda Bear and the baby panda bears. He would like you to see and play with them, so he is taking you by the hand and leading you down another path that you have not explored. The trees are bending over and murmuring welcome, and the stones and pebbles are moving out of your way so that you won't trip.

There, in front of you, is a bamboo thicket, and hidden in its midst is the panda's family. As you follow him in, you notice some colored rubber balls lying around. Why don't you pick up one? I am sure the baby pandas would love to play with you. They are like round balls of fluff themselves with little dark button eyes. Panda Bear wants you to sit on his knee while he tells the children stories. I wonder if you know these stories? Perhaps you will listen to them too . . .

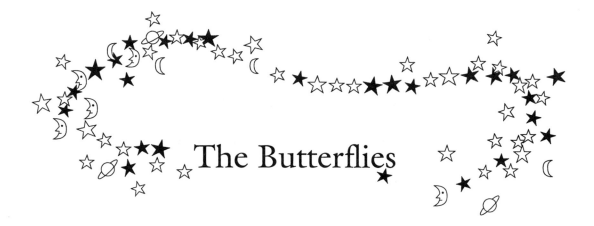

The Butterflies

THE AIR is fresh with a light breeze touching your cheek, and the sun is beaming down on you. The green grass is like a soft carpet under your feet, and the huge trees with their spreading branches are protecting the smaller plants.

As you walk down your garden path, you will notice there are lots and lots of butterflies. They are so pretty, and their colors are glorious. Do have a look at their wings, they are so fine. It's as though they had been woven by fairy threads, and then dipped into pots of paint that hold all the colors you can see in a rainbow.

Watch where the butterflies go. Can you see how busy they are with the flowers, visiting each one to say, "Hello, how are you today?" and landing very gently on their petals?

They have seen you watching them, and they are inviting you to join them in their happy task of talking to the flowers and the plants. They realize it will be difficult for you to keep up with them unless you too have wings, so Queen Butterfly is going to get you some butterfly wings and clothes that are kept near the roots of the red rose bush.

The wings being offered to you shine beautifully in the sunlight. They are of gold, black, and amber with just a tinge of silver, and the clothes are in a soft shade of yellow with little black stripes through them.

You can now take off to fly with the butterflies and see where they go. Queen Butterfly would like you to stay by her side because you are her special guest. It is her pleasure to take you to the very best flowers and shrubs in the garden.

As you fly with Queen Butterfly, you will hear all the other butterflies singing the special song they sing. They would like you to join in with them.

You will have to listen very VERY carefully . . .

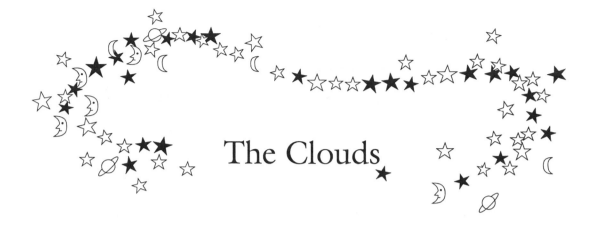

The Clouds

As YOU enter your garden, you become aware of the softness of the air caressing your cheeks, and the warmth of the sun on your body. Look around and you can see the trees and plants all sharing the same earth happily with the flowers and the animals.

The sky is a deep shade of blue although it is also very bright and clear. The golden sun is high in the heavens warming the earth and all of the earth's creatures.

The path in front of you is winding along through the soft dewy grass and up onto a hill that isn't difficult to climb. I want you to go to a soft grassy spot and lie on your back in the sun.

This way you can look at the white clouds in the sky and watch them change shape. Watch them change from little clouds to big and then back again.

Now that you are comfortable, I want you to really watch the clouds, and you will see they form very unusual shapes—if you look at them closely you might be able to see those shapes more clearly—can you see your grandpa? Or your grandma? Oh, I can see a little cat up there, and yes, there are other animals around the cat. I think it must be the cat's whole family, all together.

The clouds always keep moving and forming new shapes. Perhaps you can see whole new places that you can't see elsewhere. Sometimes you can see other lands in the sky and, way up above you, other people in these lands. Sometimes you can see mountains or buildings, or different animals. It is very peaceful watching the clouds drifting by, changing, and reappearing as something else.

Why don't you just lie there and watch, and see what else is in the sky . . .

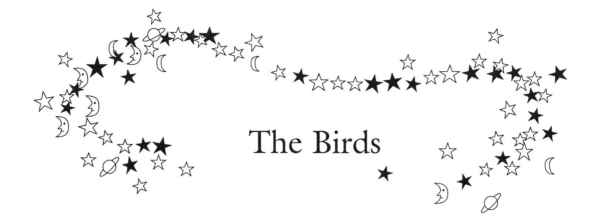

The Birds

THIS time in your garden, it is very quiet and tranquil. I can smell the scent of the flowers. The sun is high in the heavens, and the blue of the sky is light and delicate. The huge trees cast a protecting shade for the young plants, which are struggling to grow.

As you go down your garden path you will become aware of the birds calling to each other, birds of all colors and from all countries. The crow is busy laughing at the other crows, while the sparrows dart and chatter. There are plenty of parrots around screeching to each other.

There are smooth white parrots with little yellow crests on the top of their heads. These are the cockatoos. There are others that are pink, grey, and white. They are always fluffing up the feathers on their crown, and they are galahs. And there are those who are very striking indeed with their green, red, blue, orange, and yellow feathers, and they are rosellas.

Now I can see the emus coming along. They seem such funny creatures with all those feathers on their bodies, with their skinny legs and long heads. They sway along as they walk and they love having bits of bread given to them. Perhaps you could feed them by hand. I think the names of two of them are Heckle and Jeckle.

The peacock is coming now, very proudly showing off his feathers. The tail feathers make the most beautiful fan with colors of shining green and purple. The peacock loves to show off. He knows how beautiful he looks and wants everybody to look at him.

Now two white doves are circling overhead looking for a place to land. One of them has decided to use the top of your head as her landing post—she is now giving your ear a little nibble as she says "thank you" for being there.

There are many, many birds meeting in your

garden today, and each one will give you a feather to keep in remembrance of this special time.

Why don't you keep on walking so that you can see all the other birds that you haven't met yet . . .

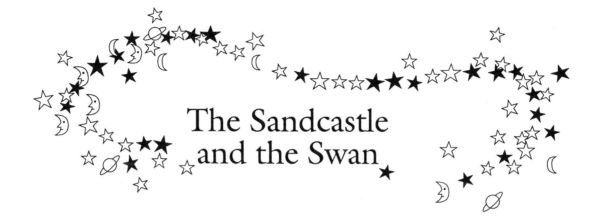

The Sandcastle
and the Swan

YOUR guardian angel is taking you down your path. You can smell the freshness of the grass. The sun is warming your body, making you feel so relaxed and at peace with the world. Feel the freshness of the air, breathe it in, and feel it cleaning your lungs.

As you go along your pathway, you will come

to a big old friendly tree that you will find near a winding river. Lean against her trunk and feel her leafy arms around you while you watch the water glistening in the sun. The water is reflecting the sun's shining rays and showing the blue of the sky in its depths.

Why don't you play in the sand near the river for a while? Perhaps you could build a sandcastle with high turrets and archways. You might need to get a little water to set the sand and to make your castle firm. Perhaps you could even put some furniture inside, and if you found a multicolored leaf, you could put it in the turret as a flag.

If you look closely you will find the sand crabs are busy scuttling across the sand. I think some of them might decide to live in your sandcastle—that is, of course, if you will let them.

Now look toward the water. You will see a white swan approaching. This swan glides along with a majestic air and is very graceful. On her back is a little wooden seat with a red velvet cushion and an umbrella over the top to shade your head from the sun's rays. If you want, you can hold the reins that lead to the swan's beak.

Why don't you step on board and sail down the river with this swan? You will have a wonderful time floating on the swan's back. Your swan will sail down the waterways, passing under the sweeping willow trees where people sometimes have picnics. As you trail your hands in the water you can push the water lilies aside, watching the ripples they make. Look into the depths of the water and you will see the golden fish swimming by . . .

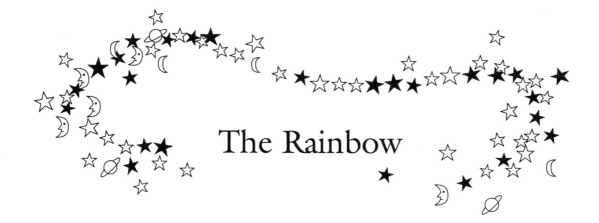

The Rainbow

IT HAS been raining in your garden, but you will find many things to do. The sun has come out again, and you can feel the warmth all around you and the peace and joy that are there. Look at the silky blue sky and the white clouds that reflect the shining golden ball that hangs in the sky. You can still see showers of silver raindrops on the leaves and grass. The flowers look as though they had been brushed by a gentle wet hand.

I want you to now look into the distance, and, as you look, you will see far, far off—a rainbow! This rainbow is very beautiful and very special. In fact, it looks as though someone painted it, because it's hard to imagine how something as glorious as this could otherwise exist.

I wonder how you will reach it? It seems a long way to walk, so I doubt you would get there for such a long time. I know. Why don't you just wish yourself there! Wishes can come true, and I am sure that if you think of the rainbow very, very hard, and wish yourself close to it, that it will happen.

So there you are, at the foot of the rainbow. Look at the colors, these are some of the colors you use in your own painting—red, yellow, green, orange, gold, silver, white, all sorts of colors.

Why don't you see what's on the other side of the rainbow? I wonder how you will get there—will you climb up? Or are there stairs? Perhaps there is an escalator to take you up and over, or perhaps you could just think very, very hard and wish yourself on the other side.

Now that you are on the far side of the rainbow, I think you should go exploring. It's very different here from the other side, isn't it? It's as beautiful as where you were but in a different way, because everything is washed gently in the rainbow's colors. But then, you are now in Rainbow Land.

Here come the Rainbow People to greet you.

Their clothing is made out of leaves in all the colors of the rainbow. Their shoes are pointed and curl in little circles over their toes. You can see their homes not very far away, but there is no need to walk there. All you have to do is *wish*.

That is what the Rainbow People do to transport themselves around.

I think I will leave you with these gentle people, as I am sure there are many things they want to show you . . .

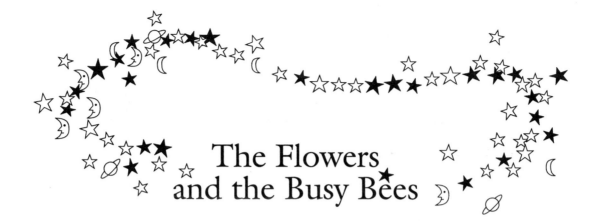

The Flowers and the Busy Bees

CAN YOU smell the scent of the flowers? Each flower has its own special aroma. Together they blend into one cloud of fragrant perfume that wafts across the fields of flowers.

You are very lucky to be in this part of the garden tonight. This is the special time when the flowers open up to those who enter, to show them their many secrets.

You can walk through these fields feeling the flowers touching you as you move. The flowers are very loving and caring, and they enjoy showing their beauty to children who treat them gently.

Look at the flowers. You notice there are many bees going about their business of gathering from the flowers the pollen to make into honey when they return to their hive. The bees are dressed in black and gold, and their wings are very fine indeed. Would you like to be a bee for a while?

Close your eyes tight and see yourself getting smaller and smaller until you are the same size as the bee. Now that you are the same size, you can see the bees are smiling at you in welcome.

They love having people visit them while they

are working. They are offering you a bee's outfit complete with wings. Put it on and you can accompany them on their journeying from flower to flower.

Now you are flitting from flower to flower. The perfume is getting stronger all the time. The bees are humming as they go about their work, and you will notice that you can hum along with them because you now feel as they do.

Do you want to explore the heart of the flower?

Look at the center of each one. You will see a little door that you could open to go inside. Why don't you say "good-bye" to the bees and return their clothing? Explain that you would like to see what is behind the flower doors.

The door in the daisy looks interesting. The knob is made out of golden mesh and the door itself is velvet. As you go inside, you find lots of activity with the Daisy People rushing to and fro to make sure that the daisy's perfume is being released properly. They are so pleased you dropped in to see them, and they would like you to stay for a while . . .

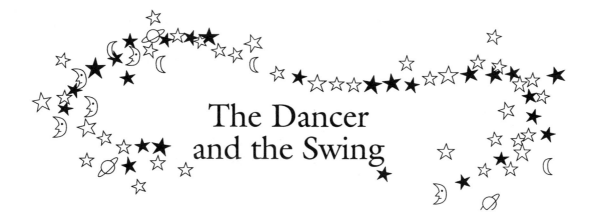

The Dancer
and the Swing

FEEL THE freshness of the air on your cheeks as you wander down your winding pathway, smelling the sweet scent from the lovely flowers that surround you.

I want you to go down the path until you come to your old wise tree. He has a present for you. Give him a big hug, and feel his energies flowing into your body making you stronger and stronger. Lean against him while he whispers into your ear, and look up into his branches, because that is where he has hidden your special present.

There, hanging from a leafy branch, are the most elegant ballet clothes you could imagine, with little pink ballet shoes alongside and a little jeweled headpiece for your hair. It is all just perfect for you, and you look very graceful as you twist and twirl around.

The rabbits and the deer are coming to watch you dance, as indeed are all the animals, as they are so fond of music. The tree is bending one of his branches over another to form a violin. The wind is whispering through the branches making music that surely must be like music made in heaven. This music makes you want to dance and dance, as though you never wanted to stop leaping and turning.

The swans are coming up the river. Their movements are making splendid formations in the water that blend with the music. Overhead the monkeys are chattering with the excitement and the pleasure of listening to the music and watching you dance. The music makes you feel as though you wanted to dance for ever and ever.

When you decide that it's time for you to rest, you will notice hanging from the wise old tree a very large swing that has a BIG, BIG bow attached to it in your favorite color, and the seat is made out of velvet and lace.

Why don't you get on the swing, and the Tree People will push you high in the air. You can feel the rush of the air past your body as you go higher and higher. You had better hold on tight though, as we wouldn't want you to fall. Even if you did fall, the grass is so soft that you wouldn't hurt yourself. Higher and higher, and that big bow is floating from the swing as the Tree People push you higher and higher. It's marvelous. You love the feeling of freedom it gives you. You can stay on the swing as long as you like . . .

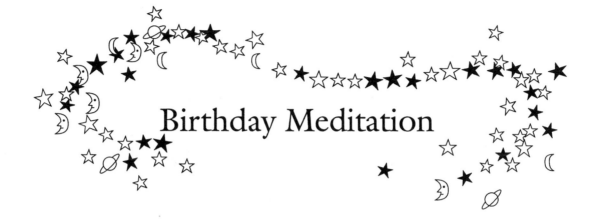

Birthday Meditation

THERE is so much joy and laughter in your garden. The birds are singing, the bees are humming, and the butterflies are darting to and fro. Look at that magnificent sky. The sun is a golden globe beaming down its warmth.

All the animals are excited, and so are the Garden People you sometimes visit. They know it's your BIRTHDAY. Birthdays are very important. On your birthday you celebrate the day of your birth, when your coming into the world brought such love and happiness to your family.

The animals are all dressed up with their fur freshly brushed and their teeth are sparkling in the sunlight. The fairies are flying from flower to flower asking them to open their petals wide in welcome. The elves are sitting on top of the mushrooms waving. The trees are nodding their branches, and their trunks are smiling in happiness as they shade the birthday cake from the sun.

And what a cake it is—big and round, with pink and yellow icing. If you look closely you can see written on it "Happy Birthday to a Special Person." Everyone is gathering around you, and they will all sing "Happy Birthday" while you blow out the candles.

The Rainbow People are putting on a special show for you with spectacular effects as they paint all the colors into a rainbow. The Cloud People are making wonderful patterns and shapes in the sky. Look how they lean over their clouds to wave and smile.

The table is laden with all of your favorite food. It is spread out on the biggest mushroom you ever saw. Everyone is looking forward to the feast, so I think you should all pull up your little shell seats, and tuck in.

But first listen, I can hear music—it's beautiful and makes you want to dance. But perhaps you should open your presents first. There is a huge pile, all very gaily wrapped in bright paper with huge red bows. I'm sure you can't wait to see what's inside . . .

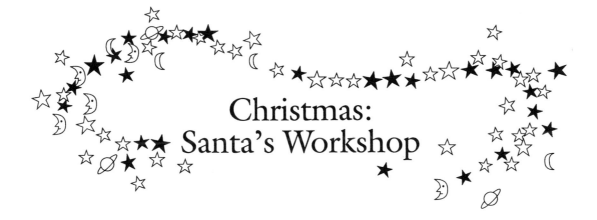

Christmas:
Santa's Workshop

THERE is so much going on in your garden tonight. I can hear all sorts of sounds, and there are different smells around also. The trees are all dressed up in tinsel and shine in the moonlight.

Each tree has a beautiful angel sitting on top. As you go along your garden path, you feel excited, for you realize it must be Christmas. I hear something! It sounds like the jingle of bells attached to a sleigh.

I wonder what on earth it could be—why it's Santa Claus! He's a very jolly old man. He is wearing a red suit and hat, and he has long white whiskers. He has come here on his sleigh with all of his eight reindeer, and they are going to take you to Santa's house, where you will meet Mrs. Claus and all of Santa's helpers.

The sleigh is very roomy and comfortable with bells fastened all the way around. There is a rug to put over your knees, because it is cold where Santa lives. When you get into the sleigh, you can sit alongside Santa and hold on tight as he takes off into the sky. You can feel the cold air on your face and hands. Santa is saying "Ho! Ho! Ho!" He is so happy to have you with him.

Now you are coming down to a faraway place all white with snow. There is Santa's house nestled away where no one could possibly find it unless they were taken there by Santa himself. It's a large white house with painted red window sills and doors. There are little turrets on top with red and green flags flying.

Santa wants you to help him select the toys for the children. He will take you to his workshop. Perhaps you could even help the elves make some. They need lots and lots of toys for all the children, especially for those children who have very few toys.

The toy shop where everything is made is wonderfully exciting. There are trains, picture puzzles, books, buses, cars, dolls, teddy bears, soft toys, dolls' houses. Whatever you could possibly imagine is there, and I really think you are going to have fun helping them make more.

When everything is finished and wrapped up in bright paper and ribbon, you will get back into the sleigh with Santa and take these toys to all the children in the world. Can you imagine their faces when they wake up and see that Santa has been? Little will they know that Santa had a very special helper this year . . .

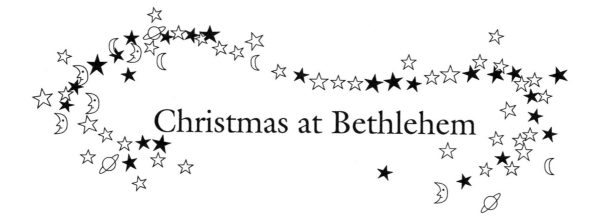

Christmas at Bethlehem

AS YOU enter your garden tonight, I want you to look at the sky. You will see a huge star, so large it's a wonder it can fit into the sky. The light from this star is streaming down upon the earth. As you look around, you will notice the birds are twittering, the rabbits are hopping, and all the animals seem to be stirring. There is a feeling tonight that something different is going to happen, something unusual and lovely.

Can you see three men coming from the eastern side of the hill? They are following the light of the star. Why don't you go with them so that you too can follow that star's brilliant light? As you join these travelers, you will notice their garments are long and flowing and brightly colored. Two of them have greying hair, while the third man's hair is silver. They all have flowing beards. They are hurrying because they know the baby Jesus is about to be born, and the light from the star is showing them the way. They will take you by the hand so that you can also share this special and blessed event. The star's light shows the way very clearly, and ahead, nestling into the hillside, is a very small building that houses animals.

The three Wise Men want you to go ahead of them through the door. They feel you should be the first person, outside the family, to see the baby who has just been born.

As you enter, you will feel the warmth the barn has to offer and smell the animals sheltering there. And there is the baby directly in front of you, being nursed by his very proud mother, Mary, and watched over by his equally proud father, Joseph. Mary and Joseph are so happy that you and the three Wise Men have come to see their new baby, and they welcome you with open arms. The baby, snuggled contentedly against his mother's sky blue dress, is smiling at you, as are Mary and Joseph.

I feel sure that if you ask them, they will allow you to nurse Jesus for a little while. Mary is holding Jesus toward you, and, as you take him into your arms and look into his eyes, you will feel a sense of unity with him, as one child to another.

The Wise Men have come with presents for the newborn baby and his parents. Do you know what your present can be? A kiss and a hug for each of them, for these are the best presents of all.

You can spend the night with this blessed family if you like. After all, it is a celebration. I know how much it would mean to you to be part of this special family . . . and so I will leave you with them . . .

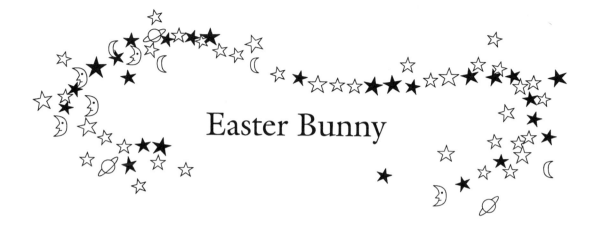

Easter Bunny

LISTEN very carefully as you enter your garden. It is very quiet. The sun is sending down its gentle rays. There are small clouds floating past catching the sun's light, which is reflecting the blue of the sky.

What can you hear? I hear movement in the bushes and I think you should go over to these bushes, but be very very quiet, as you don't want to distrub or frighten whoever it might be. Peek

through the bushes now and oh—amazing—it's
EASTER BUNNY.

He's all dressed up in his best clothes. He is
wearing a new suit that has squares all over it like a
checkerboard. A bright red hat is sitting between his
floppy ears. He has a bag in his hand—I think if you
go over to him and say "excuse me" so you don't
alarm him, he might let you look in his bag.

The bag is very big and very heavy. I wonder
what it holds? Easter eggs!! How terrific! He is
going to hide them in the garden so that everyone
can have a treasure hunt, but because the bag is so
heavy and full, he would like you to help him.

There is a small bag there for you that you can
load up with Easter eggs that you can hide from the

children. It will be such fun hiding the eggs. You could put them under flowers, in rabbit hutches, high in trees, in the tall grass, wherever you like.

Now that all the Easter eggs are hidden, Easter Bunny is going to blow his whistle, and the other children can come to where you are in the garden to start searching. They are so excited as they start looking. They are even more excited when they find these brightly colored eggs.

Mrs. Easter Bunny is coming along now with the rabbit children. They are very happy that everyone is having such a good time. She's inviting you all back to their hutch for some music and some soft drinks. They also plan on playing lots of games, so I think you should wander along with them too . . .

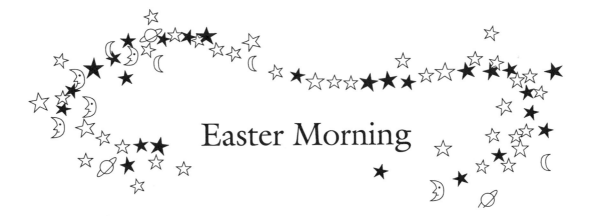

Easter Morning

YOU CAN feel something quite exciting is going to happen in your garden tonight. There is a stillness in the air, a hushed feeling of expectancy as though no one were quite sure of what is coming.

Keep walking down your garden path, as you always do, stopping to talk to the trees and the animals on the way, until you come to a hillside where a huge brown rock appears to be blocking the entrance to a cave.

If you wait a little while, you will see other people coming to join you. You might not understand why their faces are sad as they look at the rock, which appears to be immovable. If you listen very quietly, you will hear the sound of the rock scraping on the ground—indeed, I think you will hear it way before the other people. Yes, the rock is moving. That huge, heavy rock that would take many people to shift is moving on its own.

As it moves, you can see the entrance to the cave, and you will notice that the inside is lit as if by magic lanterns. A slender man with flowing garments is coming out from this cave to where you are standing, and he is bringing the light with him.

As you look, you will see the light is coming from all over his body as he stands there with his arms outstretched. This is Jesus, who has risen from the dead. Jesus would like to embrace you and to bring his light around you. He wants you to understand that there is no death; that the spirit lives on, and that he is always with you. He is taking you by the hand and leading you and the others into the town so that the people there can see the beauty of his light and his being. Why don't you go with him? He is smiling down at you. He is happy to have your hand in his and to take you with him . . .